MW01232440

The Super-Fast Ketogenic Diet Cookbook

Quick and Tasty Air Fryer Snacks Recipes to Stay
Healthy and Boost Your Brain

America Keto Recipes

Table of Contents

1. Cauliflower with Buffalo Sauce 5

2. Cheesy Bacon-Wrapped Jalapeño 8

3. Prosciutto Cheese Asparagus Roll 10

4. Cheesy Mushroom 12

5. Three Cheese Dip 14

6. Cheese Chicken Dip 16

7. Beef and Bacon Cheese Dip 18

8. Cheesy Spinach Artichoke Dip 20

9. Cheesy Pizza Crust 22

10. Sausage and Bacon Cheese Pizza 24

11. Air Fried Almond 26

12. Cheesy Chicken with Bacon 28

13. Beef Jerky 30

14. Pepperoni Cheese Roll 32

15. Spinach Turkey Meatball 34

16. Cheesy Calamari Rings 36

17. Bacon-Wrapped Onion Rings 38

18. Bacon-Wrapped Cabbage Bites 40

19. Cheesy Chicken Wings 42

20. Air Fried Chicken Wings 44

21. Golden Pork Egg 47

22. Bacon Jalapeño Cheese Bread 49

23. Cheesy Bacon Pepper 51

24. Prosciutto-Wrapped Guacamole Rings 53

25. Cheesy Pork Rind Tortillas 56

26. Cheesy Pork and Chicken 58

27.Pork Cheese Sticks 60

28.Cheesy Cauliflower Buns... 62

29.Bacon Cauliflower Skewers 64

30.Crispy Cheese Salami Roll-Ups 66

31.Cheesy Zucchini Fries 68

32.Aromatic Avocado Fries 70

33.Cheesy Pickle Spear.. 73

34.Crispy Pepperoni Chips... 75

35.Vinegary Pork Belly Chips 77

36.Air Fried Kale Chips 79

37.Prosciutto Pierogi 81

38.Air Fried Brussels Sprout 84

39.Savory Eggplant... 86

40.Golden Cheese Crisps 88

41.Broccoli Fries with Spicy Dip.................................... 90

42.Cheesy Broccoli... 92

43.Spinach Melts with Chilled Sauce 94

44.Aromatic Bacon Shrimp 97

45.Roasted Zucchini.. 99

46.Cheesy Meatball.. 101

47.Pork Meatball.. 103

48.Beef Cheese Burger 105

49.Cheesy Chicken Nuggets 107

50.Crisp Cauliflower 109

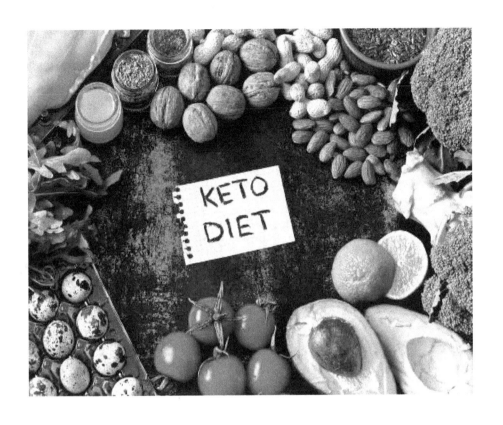

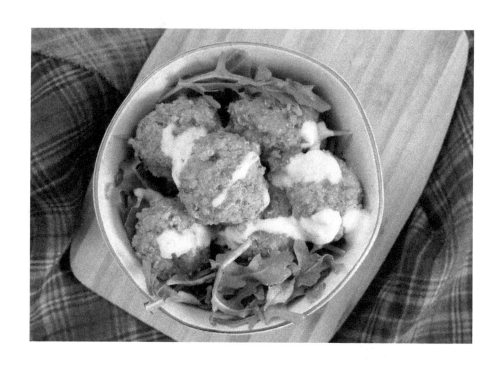

1. Cauliflower with Buffalo Sauce

Prep Time:5 m | **Cook time:**15 m | **Serves:** 6

- 1 medium head cauliflower, leaves and core removed, cut into bite-sized pieces
- 4 tablespoons salted butter, melted
- ¼ cup dry ranch seasoning
- ⅓ cup sugar-free buffalo sauce

1. Place cauliflower pieces into a large bowl. Pour butter over the cauliflower and toss to coat. Sprinkle in ranch seasoning and toss to coat.
2. Place cauliflower into an ungreased air fryer basket. Adjust the temperature to 350°F (180ºC) and set the timer for 12 minutes, shaking the basket three times during cooking.
3. When timer beeps, place cooked cauliflower in a large clean bowl. Toss with buffalo sauce, then return to air fryer basket to cook for another 3 minutes. Cauliflower bites will be darkened at the edges and tender when done.

Per Serving: calories: 112 | fat: 7g | protein: 2g | carbs: 9g | net carbs: 7g | fiber: 2g

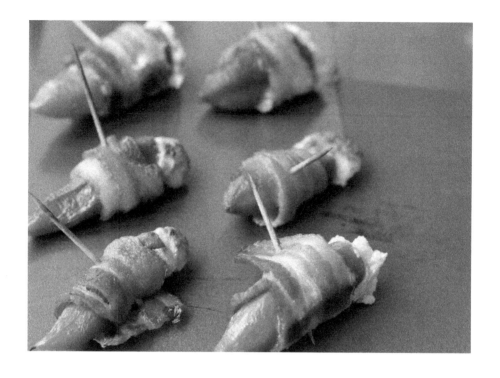

2.Cheesy Bacon-Wrapped Jalapeño

Prep Time:10 m | **Cook time:**12 m | Makes 12 poppers

- 3 ounces (85 g) cream cheese, softened ⅓ cup shredded mild Cheddar cheese
- ¼ teaspoon garlic powder
- 6 jalapeños (approximately 4-inch long), tops removed, sliced in half lengthwise, and seeded
- 12 slices sugar-free bacon

1. Place cream cheese, Cheddar, and garlic powder in a large microwave-safe bowl. Microwave 30 seconds on high, then stir. Spoon cheese mixture evenly into hollowed jalapeños.
2. Wrap 1 slice of bacon around each jalapeño half, completely covering jalapeño, and secure with a toothpick. Place jalapeños into an ungreased air fryer basket. Adjust the temperature to 400°F (205ºC) and set the timer for 12 minutes, turning jalapeños halfway through cooking. Bacon will be crispy when done.

Per Serving: calories: 278 | fat: 21g | protein: 15g | carbs: 3g | net carbs: 2g | fiber: 1g

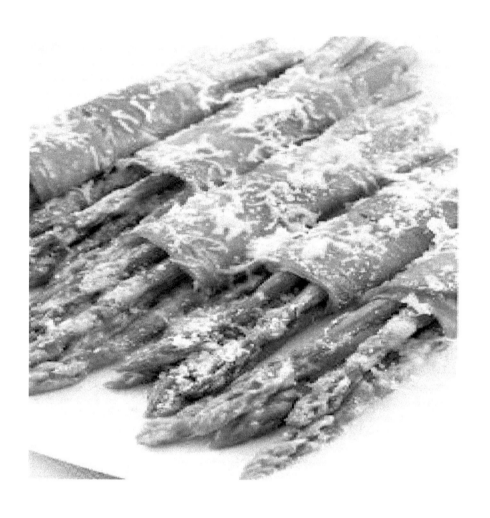

3.Prosciutto Cheese Asparagus Roll

Prep Time:10 m | **Cook time:**10 m | **Serves:** 4

- 1 pound (454 g) asparagus
- 12 (0.5-ounce 14-g) slices prosciutto
- 1 tablespoon coconut oil, melted
- 2 teaspoons lemon juice
- ⅛ teaspoon red pepper flakes ⅓ cup grated Parmesan cheese
- 2 tablespoons salted butter, melted

1. On a clean work surface, place an asparagus spear onto a slice of prosciutto.
2. Drizzle with coconut oil and lemon juice. Sprinkle red pepper flakes and Parmesan across asparagus. Roll prosciutto around an asparagus spear. Place into the air fryer basket.
3. Adjust the temperature to 375°F (190ºC) and set the timer for 10 minutes.
4. Drizzle the asparagus roll with butter before serving.

Per Serving: calories: 263 | fat: 20g | protein: 14g | carbs: 7g | net carbs: 4g | fiber: 3g

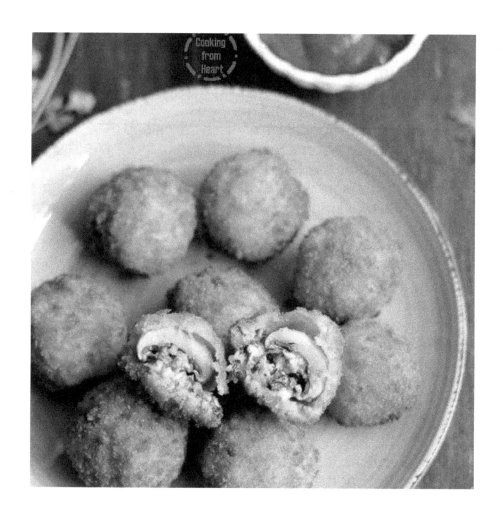

4.Cheesy Mushroom

Prep Time:10 m | **Cook time:**8 m | **Serves:** 20 mushrooms

- 4 ounces (113 g) cream cheese, softened
- 6 tablespoons shredded pepper jack cheese
- 2 tablespoons chopped pickled jalapeños
- 20 medium button mushrooms, stems removed
- 2 tablespoons olive oil
- ¼ teaspoon salt
- ⅛ teaspoon ground black pepper

1. In a large bowl, mix cream cheese, pepper jack, and jalapeños.
2. Drizzle mushrooms with olive oil, then sprinkle with salt and pepper. Spoon 2 tablespoons cheese mixture into each mushroom and place in a single layer into an ungreased air fryer basket. Adjust the temperature to 370°F (188ºC) and set the timer for 8 minutes, checking halfway through cooking to ensure even cooking, rearranging if some are darker than others. When they're golden and cheese is bubbling, mushrooms will be done.

Per Serving: calories: 87 | fat: 7g | protein: 3g | carbs: 2g | net carbs: 2g | fiber: 0g

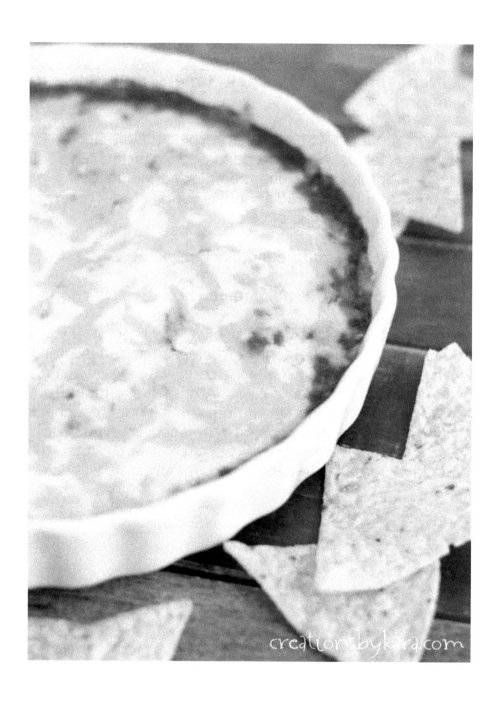

creationsbykira.com

5.Three Cheese Dip

Prep Time:5 m | **Cook time:**12 m | **Serves:** 8

- 8 ounces (227 g) cream cheese, softened
- ½ cup mayonnaise ¼ cup sour cream
- ½ cup shredded sharp Cheddar cheese ¼ cup shredded Monterey jack cheese

1. In a large bowl, combine all ingredients. Scoop mixture into an ungreased 4-cup nonstick baking dish and place into air fryer basket.
2. Adjust the temperature to 375°F (190°C) and set the timer for 12 minutes. Dip will be browned on top and bubbling when done. Serve warm.

Per Serving: calories: 245 | fat: 23g | protein: 5g | carbs: 2g | net carbs: 2g | fiber: 0g

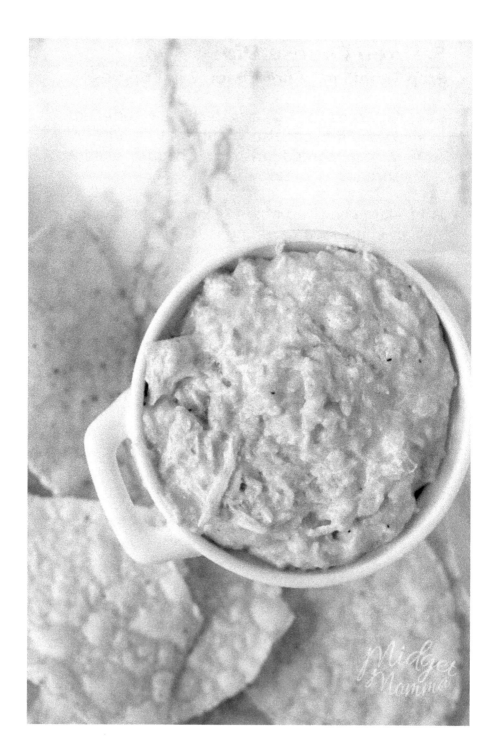

6.Cheese Chicken Dip

Prep Time:10 m | **Cook time:**12 m | **Serves:** 8

- 8 ounces (227 g) cream cheese, softened
- 2 cups chopped cooked chicken thighs
- ½ cup sugar-free buffalo sauce
- 1 cup shredded mild Cheddar cheese, divided

1. In a large bowl, combine cream cheese, chicken, buffalo sauce, and ½ cup Cheddar. Scoop the dip into an ungreased 4-cup nonstick baking dish and top with remaining Cheddar.
2. Place dish into air fryer basket. Adjust the temperature to 375°F (190ºC) and set the timer for 12 minutes. The dip will be browned on top and bubbling when done. Serve warm.

Per Serving: calories: 222 | fat: 15g | protein: 14g | carbs:1g | net carbs: 1g | fiber: 0g

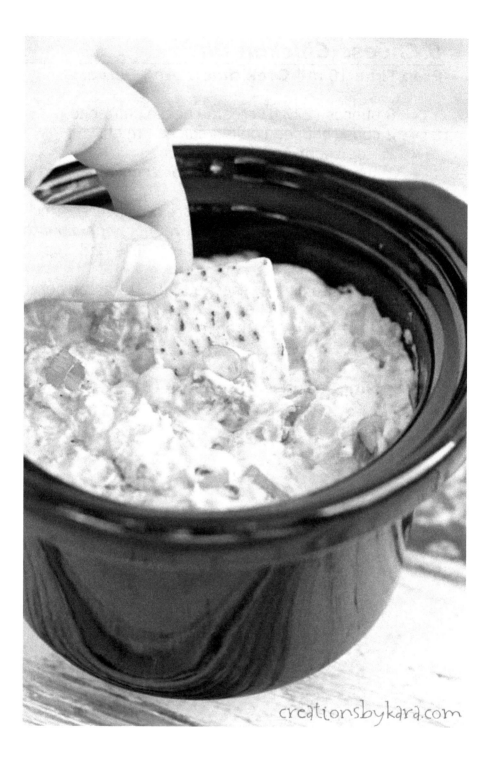

7.Beef and Bacon Cheese Dip

Prep Time:20 m | **Cook time:**10 m | **Serves:** 6

- 8 ounces (227 g) full-fat cream cheese
- ¼ cup full-fat mayonnaise
- ¼ cup full-fat sour cream
- ¼ cup chopped onion
- 1 teaspoon garlic powder
- 1 tablespoon Worcestershire sauce
- 1¼ cups shredded medium Cheddar cheese, divided
- ½ pound (227g) cooked 80/20 ground beef
- 6 slices sugar-free bacon, cooked and crumbled
- 2 large pickle spears, chopped

1. Place cream cheese in a large microwave-safe bowl and microwave for 45 seconds. Stir in mayonnaise, sour cream, onion, garlic powder, Worcestershire sauce, and 1 cup Cheddar. Add cooked ground beef and bacon. Sprinkle remaining Cheddar on top.
2. Place in a 6-inch bowl and put into the air fryer basket.
3. Adjust the temperature to 400°F (205ºC) and set the timer for 10 minutes.
4. Dip is done when the top is golden and bubbling. Sprinkle pickles over the dish. Serve warm.

Per Serving: calories: 457 | fat: 35g | protein: 22g | carbs: 4g | net carbs: 3g | fiber: 1g

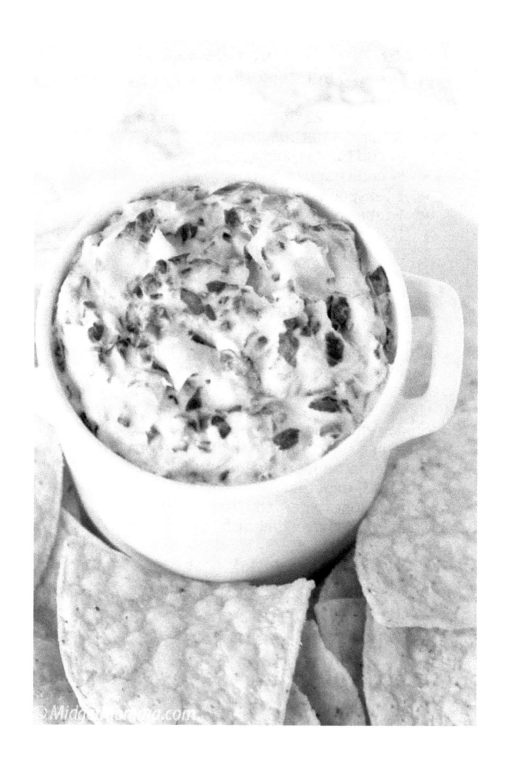

8. Cheesy Spinach Artichoke Dip

Prep Time: 10 m | **Cook time:** 10 m | **Serves:** 6

- 10 ounces (283 g) frozen spinach, drained and thawed
- 1 (14-ounce / 397-g) can artichoke hearts, drained and chopped ¼ cup chopped pickled jalapeños
- 8 ounces (227 g) full-fat cream cheese, softened
- ¼ cup full-fat mayonnaise
- ¼ cup full-fat sour cream ½ teaspoon garlic powder
- ¼ cup grated Parmesan cheese
- 1 cup shredded pepper jack cheese

1. Mix all ingredients in a 4-cup baking bowl. Place into the air fryer basket.
2. Adjust the temperature to 320°F (160ºC) and set the timer for 10 minutes.
3. Remove when brown and bubbling. Serve warm.

Per Serving: calories: 226 | fat: 15g | protein: 10g | carbs: 10g | net carbs: 6g | fiber: 4g

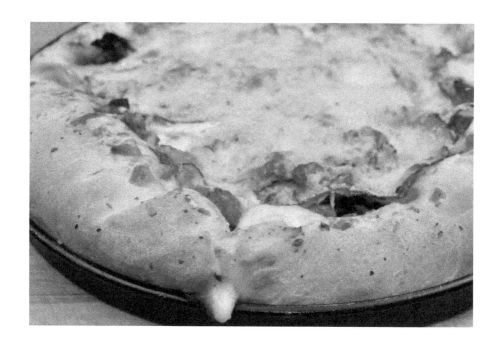

9.Cheesy Pizza Crust

Prep Time:5 m | **Cook time:**10 m | **Serves:** 1

- ½ cup shredded whole-milk Mozzarella cheese
- 2 tablespoons blanched finely ground almond flour
- 1 tablespoon full-fat cream cheese
- 1 large egg white

1. Place Mozzarella, almond flour, and cream cheese in a medium microwave-safe bowl. Microwave for 30 seconds. Stir until a smooth ball of dough forms. Add egg white and stir until soft round dough forms.
2. Press into a 6-inch round pizza crust.
3. Cut a piece of parchment to fit your air fryer basket and place crust on parchment. Place into the air fryer basket.
4. Adjust the temperature to 350°F (180ºC) and set the timer for 10 minutes.
5. Flip after 5 minutes, and at this time, place any desired toppings on the crust. Continue cooking until golden.
Per Serving: calories: 314 | fat: 22g | protein: 20g | carbs: 5g | net carbs: 3g | fiber: 2g

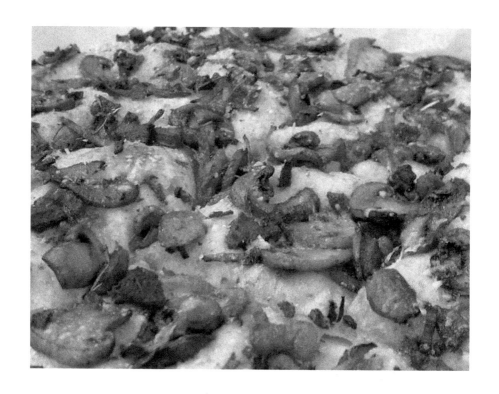

10.Sausage and Bacon Cheese Pizza

Prep Time:5 m | **Cook time:**5 m | **Serves:** 1

- ½ cup shredded Mozzarella cheese
- 7 slices pepperoni
- ¼ cup cooked ground sausage
- 2 slices sugar-free bacon, cooked and crumbled
- 1 tablespoon grated Parmesan cheese
- 2 tablespoons low-carb, sugar-free pizza sauce for dipping

1. Cover the bottom of a 6-inch cake pan with Mozzarella. Place pepperoni, sausage, and bacon on top of the cheese and sprinkle with Parmesan. Place pan into the air fryer basket.
2. Adjust the temperature to 400°F (205ºC) and set the timer for 5 minutes.
3. Remove when the cheese is bubbling and golden. Serve warm with pizza sauce for dipping.

Per Serving: calories: 466 | fat: 34g | protein: 28g | carbs: 5g | net carbs: 4g | fiber: 1g

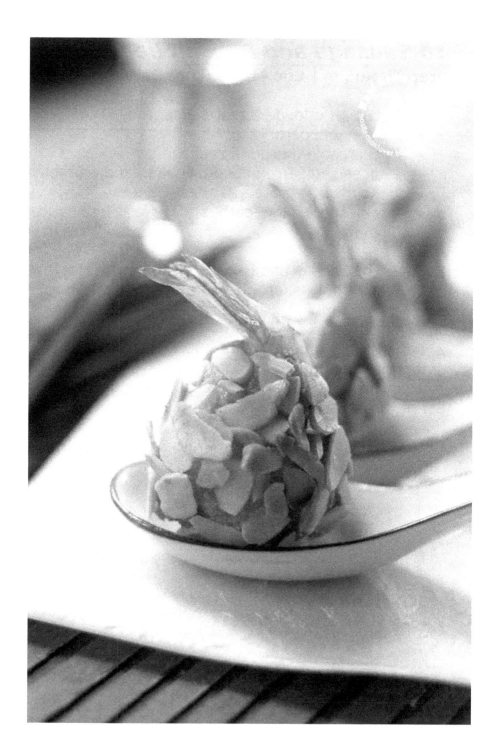

11.Air Fried Almond

Prep time: 5 m | **Cook time:**6 m | **Serves:** 4

- 1 cup raw almonds
- 2 teaspoons coconut oil
- 1 teaspoon chili powder
- ¼ teaspoon cumin
- ¼ teaspoon smoked paprika
- ¼ teaspoon onion powder

1. In a large bowl, toss all ingredients until almonds are evenly coated with oil and spices. Place almonds into the air fryer basket.
2. Adjust the temperature to 320°F (160ºC) and set the timer for 6 minutes.
3. Toss the fryer basket halfway through the cooking time. Allow cooling completely.

Per Serving: calories: 182 | fat: 16g | protein: 6g | carbs: 7g | net carbs: 3g | fiber: 4g

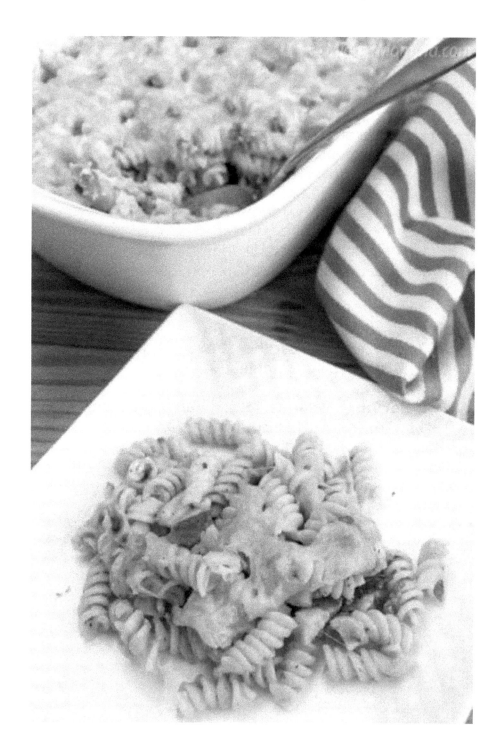

12.Cheesy Chicken with Bacon

Prep Time:10 m | **Cook time:**15 m | **Serves:** 6

- 2 (6-ounce / 170-g) boneless, skinless chicken breasts, cut into 1-inch cubes
- 1 tablespoon coconut oil
- ½ teaspoon salt
- ¼ teaspoon ground black pepper ⅓ cup ranch dressing
- ½ cup shredded Colby cheese
- 4 slices cooked sugar-free bacon, crumbled

1. Drizzle chicken with coconut oil. Sprinkle with salt and pepper, and place into an ungreased 6-inch round nonstick baking dish.
2. Place dish into air fryer basket. Adjust the temperature to 370°F (188ºC) and set the timer for 10 minutes, stirring chicken halfway through cooking.
3. When the timer beeps, drizzle ranch dressing over chicken and top with Colby and bacon. Adjust the temperature to 400°F (205ºC) and set the timer for 5 minutes. When done, the chicken will be browned and have an internal temperature of at least 165°F (74ºC).

Per Serving: calories: 164 | fat: 9g | protein: 18g | carbs: 0g | net carbs: 0g | fiber: 0g

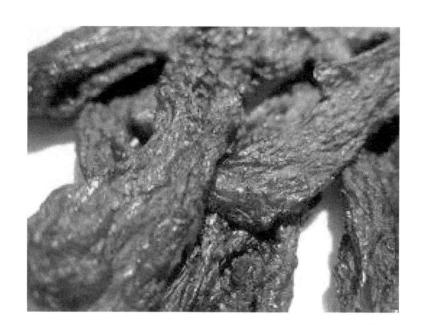

13.Beef Jerky

Prep Time:5 m | **Cook time:**4 ho | **Serves:** 10

- 1 pound (454 g) flat iron beef, thinly sliced ¼ cup coconut aminos
- 2 teaspoons Worcestershire sauce
- ¼ teaspoon crushed red pepper flakes
- ¼ teaspoon garlic powder
- ¼ teaspoon onion powder

1. Place all ingredients into a plastic storage bag or covered container and marinate for 2 hours in the refrigerator.
2. Place each slice of jerky on the air fryer rack in a single layer.
3. Adjust the temperature to 160°F (71ºC) and set the timer for 4 hours.
4. Cool and store in an airtight container for up to 1 week.

Per Serving: calories: 85 | fat: 3g | protein: 10g | carbs: 1g | net carbs: 1g | fiber: 0g

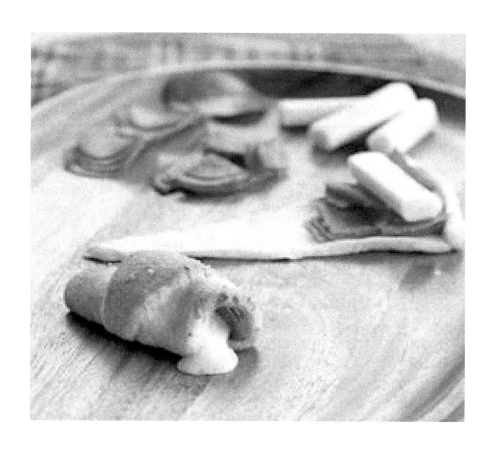

14. Pepperoni Cheese Roll

Prep time: 5 m | **Cook time:** 8 m | Makes 12 rolls

- 2½ cups shredded Mozzarella cheese
- 2 ounces (57 g) cream cheese, softened
- 1 cup blanched finely ground almond flour
- 48 slices pepperoni
- 2 teaspoons Italian seasoning

1. In a large microwave-safe bowl, combine Mozzarella, cream cheese, and flour. Microwave on high for 90 seconds until cheese is melted.
2. Using a wooden spoon, mix melted mixture 2 minutes until a dough forms.
3. Once the dough is cool enough to work with your hands, about 2 minutes, spread it out into a 12-inch × 4-inch rectangle on ungreased parchment paper. Line dough with pepperoni, divided into four even rows. Sprinkle Italian seasoning evenly over pepperoni.
4. Starting at the long end of the dough, roll up until a log is formed. Slice the log into twelve even pieces.
5. Place pizza rolls in an ungreased 6-inch nonstick baking dish. Adjust the temperature to 375°F (190ºC) and set the timer for 8 minutes. Rolls will be golden and firm when done. Allow cooked rolls to cool 10 minutes before serving.

Per Serving: calories: 366 | fat: 27g | protein: 20g | carbs: 7g | net carbs: 5g | fiber: 2g

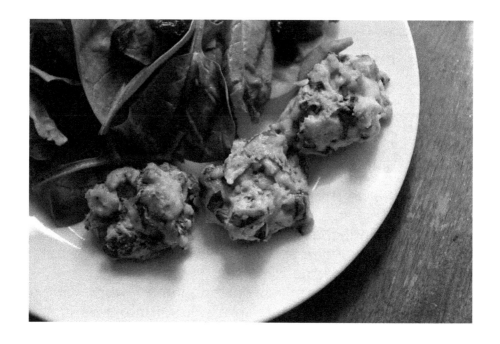

15.Spinach Turkey Meatball

Prep Time:10 m | **Cook time:**10 m | **Makes** 36 meatballs

- 1 cup fresh spinach leaves
- ¼ cup peeled and diced red onion ½ cup crumbled feta cheese
- 1 pound (454 g) 85/15 ground turkey ½ teaspoon salt
- ½ teaspoon ground cumin
- ¼ teaspoon ground black pepper

1. Place spinach, onion, and feta in a food processor, and pulse ten times until spinach is chopped. Scoop into a large bowl.

2. Add turkey to the bowl and sprinkle with salt, cumin, and pepper. Mix until thoroughly combined. Roll mixture into thirty-six meatballs (about 1 tablespoon each).

3. Place meatballs into an ungreased air fryer basket, working in batches if needed. Adjust the temperature to 350°F (180ºC) and set the timer for 10 minutes, shaking the basket twice during cooking. Meatballs will be browned and have an internal temperature of at least 165°F (74ºC) when done. Serve warm.

Per Serving: calories: 115 | fat: 7g | protein: 10g | carbs: 1g | net carbs: 1g | fiber: 0g

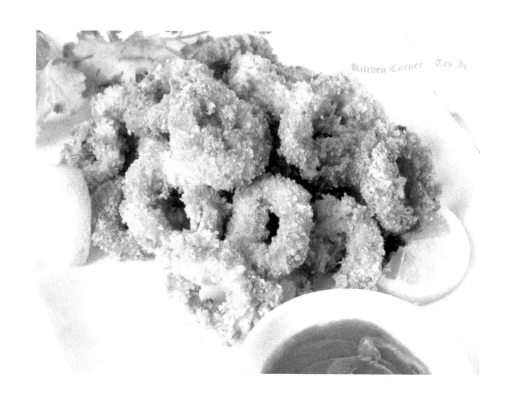

Kitchen Corner - Try It

16.Cheesy Calamari Rings

Prep Time:10 m | **Cook time:**15 m | **Serves:** 4

- 2 large egg yolks
- 1 cup powdered Parmesan cheese (or pork dust for dairy-free; see here)
- ¼ cup coconut flour
- 3 teaspoons dried oregano leaves
- ½ teaspoon garlic powder
- ½ teaspoon onion powder
- 1 pound (454 g) calamari, sliced into rings
- Fresh oregano leaves for garnish (optional)
- 1 cup no-sugar-added marinara sauce, for serving (optional)
- Lemon slices, for serving (optional)

1. Spray the air fryer basket with avocado oil. Preheat the air fryer to 400°F (205ºC).
2. In a shallow dish, whisk the egg yolks. In a separate bowl, mix the Parmesan, coconut flour, and spices.
3. Dip the calamari rings in the egg yolks, tap off any excess egg, then dip them into the cheese mixture and coat well. Use your hands to press the coating onto the calamari if necessary. Spray the coated rings with avocado oil.
4. Place the calamari rings in the air fryer, leaving space between them, and cook for 15 minutes or until golden brown. If desired, garnish with fresh oregano, and serve with a marinara sauce for dipping and lemon slices.
5. Best served fresh. Store leftovers in an airtight container in the fridge for up to 5 days. Reheat in a preheated 400°F (205ºC) air fryer for 3 minutes or until heated through.

Per Serving: calories: 287 | fat: 13g | protein: 28g | carbs: 11g | net carbs: 8g | fiber: 3g

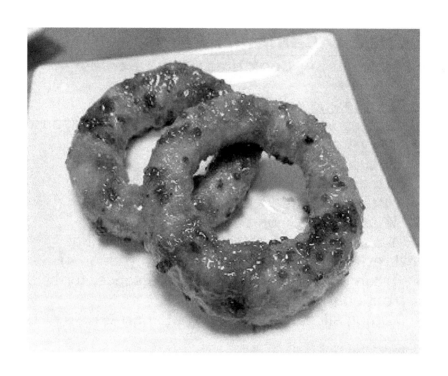

17.Bacon-Wrapped Onion Rings

Prep Time:5 m | **Cook time:**10 m | **Serves:** 8

- 1 large white onion, peeled and cut into 16 (¼-inch-thick) slices
- 8 slices sugar-free bacon

1. Stack 2 slices of onion and wrap with 1 slice of bacon. Secure with a toothpick. Repeat with remaining onion slices and bacon.
2. Place onion rings into an ungreased air fryer basket. Adjust the temperature to 350°F (180ºC) and set the timer for 10 minutes, turning rings halfway through cooking. Bacon will be crispy when done. Serve warm.

Per Serving: calories: 84 | fat: 4g | protein: 5g | carbs: 8g | net carbs: 6g | fiber: 2g

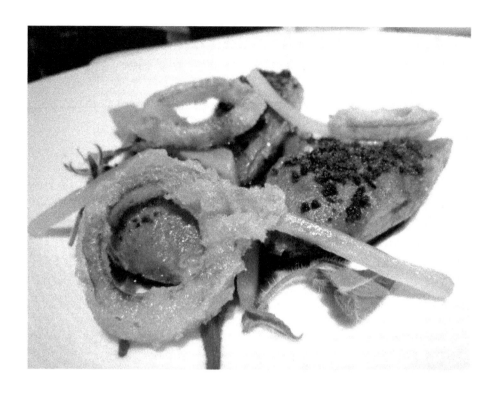

18.Bacon-Wrapped Cabbage Bites

Prep Time:10 m | **Cook time:**12 m | **Serves:** 6

- 3 tablespoons sriracha hot chili sauce, divided
- 1 medium head cabbage, cored and cut into 12 bite-sized pieces
- 2 tablespoons coconut oil, melted
- ½ teaspoon salt
- 12 slices sugar-free bacon
- ½ cup mayonnaise
- ¼ teaspoon garlic powder

1. Evenly brush 2 tablespoons of sriracha onto cabbage pieces. Drizzle evenly with coconut oil, then sprinkle with salt.
2. Wrap each cabbage piece with bacon and secure with a toothpick. Place into an ungreased air fryer basket. Adjust the temperature to 375°F (190ºC) and set the timer for 12 minutes, turning cabbage halfway through cooking. Bacon will be cooked and crispy when done.
3. In a small bowl, whisk together mayonnaise, garlic powder, and remaining sriracha. Use as a dipping sauce for cabbage bites.

Per Serving: calories: 316 | fat: 26g | protein: 10g | carbs: 11g | net carbs: 7g | fiber: 4g

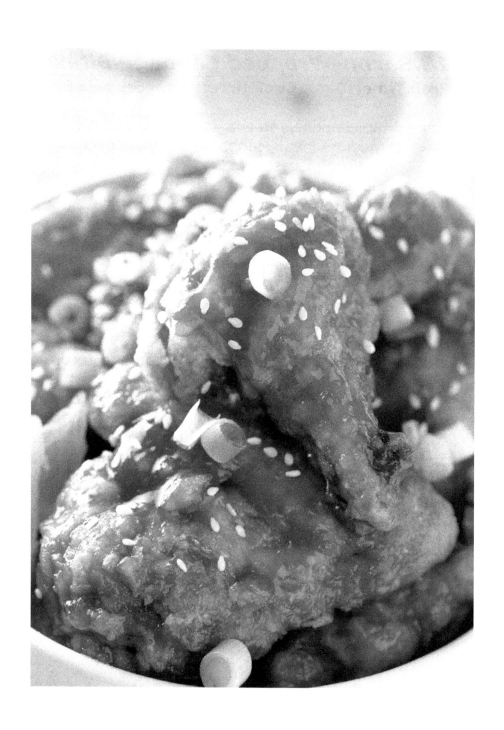

19. Cheesy Chicken Wings

Prep Time: 5 m | **Cook time:** 25 m | **Serves:** 4

- 2 pounds (907 g) raw chicken wings
- 1 teaspoon pink Himalayan salt
- ½ teaspoon garlic powder
- 1 tablespoon baking powder
- 4 tablespoons unsalted butter, melted $1/3$ cup grated Parmesan cheese
- ¼ teaspoon dried parsley

1. In a large bowl, place chicken wings, salt, ½ teaspoon garlic powder, baking powder, and then toss. Place wings into the air fryer basket.
2. Adjust the temperature to 400°F (205ºC) and set the timer for 25 minutes.
3. Toss the basket two or three times during the cooking time.
4. In a small bowl, combine butter, Parmesan, and parsley.
5. Remove wings from the fryer and place them into a large clean bowl. Pour the butter mixture over the wings and toss until coated. Serve warm.

Per Serving: calories: 565 | fat: 42g | protein: 42g | carbs: 2g | net carbs: 2g | fiber: 0g

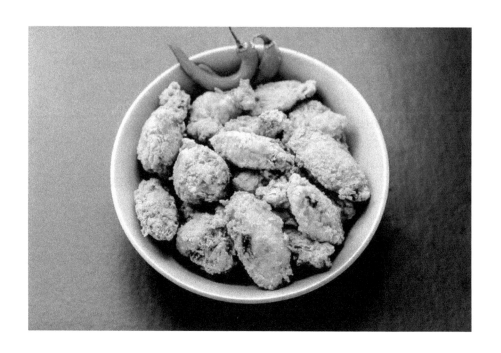

20.Air Fried Chicken Wings

Prep Time:5 m | **Cook time:**32 m | **Serves:** 1 dozen wings

- 1 dozen chicken wings or drummies
- 1 tablespoon coconut oil or bacon fat, melted
- 2 teaspoons berbere spice
- 1 teaspoon acceptable sea salt

For Serving
- (Omit For Egg-Free):
- 2 hard-boiled eggs
- ½ teaspoon fine sea salt ¼ teaspoon berbere spice ¼ teaspoon dried chives

1. Spray the air fryer basket with avocado oil. Preheat the air fryer to 380°F (193ºC).
2. Place the chicken wings in a large bowl. Pour the oil over them and turn to coat thoroughly. Sprinkle the berbere and salt on all sides of the chicken.
3. Place the chicken wings in the air fryer and cook for 25 minutes, flipping after 15 minutes.
4. After 25 minutes, increase the temperature to 400°F (205ºC) and cook for 6 to 7 minutes more until the skin is browned and crisp.
5. While the chicken cooks, prepare the hard-boiled eggs (if using): Peel the eggs, slice them in half, and season them with the salt, berbere, and dried chives. Serve the chicken and eggs together.
6. Store leftovers in an airtight container in the fridge for up to 4 days. Reheat the chicken in a preheated 400°F (205ºC) air fryer for 5 minutes or until heated through.

Per Serving: calories: 317 | fat: 24g | protein: 24g | carbs: 1g | net carbs: 1g | fiber: 0g

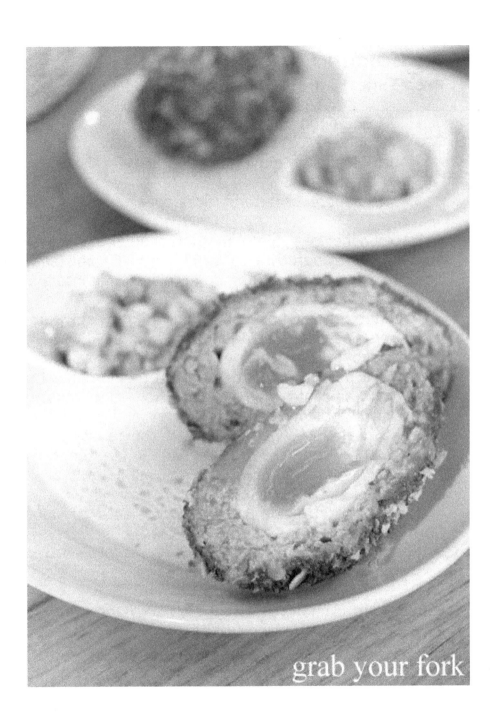

grab your fork

21.Golden Pork Egg

Prep Time:10 m | **Cook time:**25 m | Makes 12 eggs

- 7 large eggs, divided
- 1 ounce (28 g) plain pork rinds, finely crushed
- 2 tablespoons mayonnaise
- ¼ teaspoon salt
- ¼ teaspoon ground black pepper

1. Place 6 whole eggs into an ungreased air fryer basket. Adjust the temperature to 220°F (104ºC) and set the timer for 20 minutes. When done, place eggs into a bowl of ice water to cool for 5 minutes.
2. Peel cool eggs, then cut in half lengthwise. Remove yolks and place them aside in a medium bowl.
3. In a separate small bowl, whisk the remaining raw egg. Place pork rinds in a separate medium bowl. Dip each egg white into whisked egg, then gently coat with pork rinds. Spritz with cooking spray and place into an ungreased air fryer basket. Adjust the temperature to 400°F (205ºC) and set the timer for 5 minutes, turning eggs halfway through cooking. Eggs will be golden when done.
4. Mash yolks in a bowl with mayonnaise until smooth. Sprinkle with salt and pepper and mix.
5. Spoon 2 tablespoons of yolk mixture into each fried egg white.

Per Serving: calories: 141 | fat: 10g | protein: 10g | carbs: 1g | net carbs: 1g | fiber: 0g

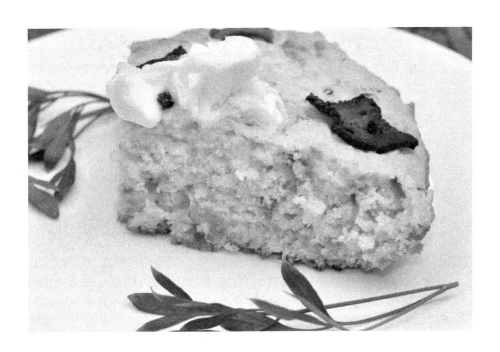

22.Bacon Jalapeño Cheese Bread

Prep Time:10 m | **Cook time:**15 m | **Serves:** 8

- 2 cups shredded Mozzarella cheese
- ¼ cup grated Parmesan cheese
- ¼ cup chopped pickled jalapeños
- 2 large eggs
- 4 slices sugar-free bacon, cooked and chopped

1. Mix all ingredients in a large bowl. Cut a piece of parchment to fit your air fryer basket.
2. Dampen your hands with a bit of water and press out the mixture into a circle. You may need to separate this into two smaller cheese bread, depending on your fryer's size.
3. Place the parchment and cheese bread into the air fryer basket.
4. Adjust the temperature to 320°F (160ºC) and set the timer for 15 minutes.
5. Carefully flip the bread when 5 minutes remain.
6. When fully cooked, the top will be golden brown.

Per Serving: calories: 273 | fat: 18g | protein: 20g | carbs: 3g | net carbs: 2g | fiber: 1g

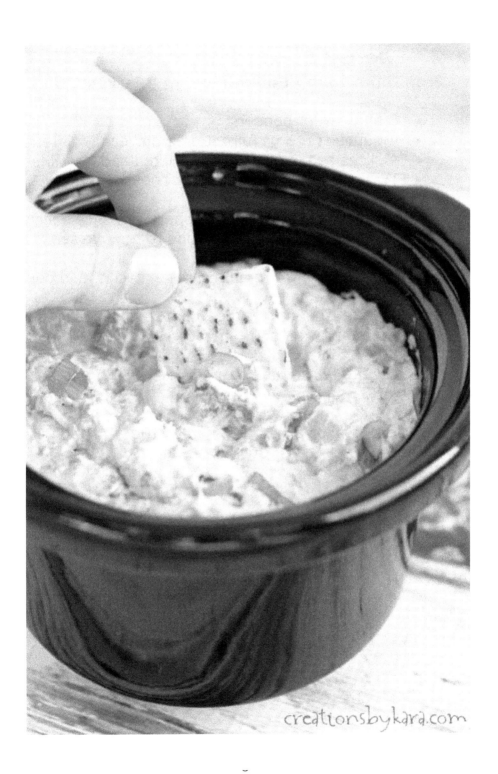

creationsbykara.com

23.Cheesy Bacon Pepper

Prep time: 15 m | **Cook time:**8 m | **Serves:** 16

- 8 mini sweet peppers
- 4 ounces (113 g) full-fat cream cheese, softened
- 4 slices sugar-free bacon, cooked and crumbled
- ¼ cup shredded pepper jack cheese

1. Remove the tops from the peppers and slice each one in half lengthwise. Use a small knife to remove seeds and membranes.
2. In a small bowl, mix cream cheese, bacon, and pepper jack.
3.Place 3 teaspoons of the mixture into each sweet pepper and press down smooth. Place into the fryer basket.
4. Adjust the temperature to 400°F (205ºC) and set the timer for 8 minutes.

Per Serving: calories: 176 | fat: 13g | protein: 7g | carbs: 4g | net carbs: 3g | fiber: 1g

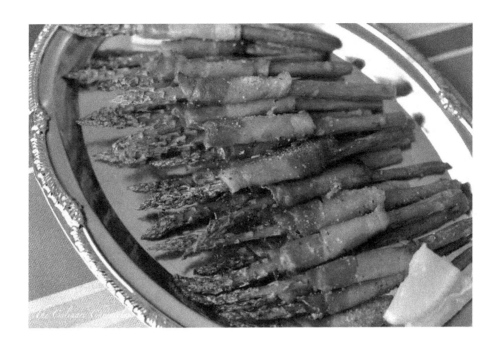

24.Prosciutto-Wrapped Guacamole Rings

Prep time: 10 m | **Cook time:**6 m | **Makes** 8 rings

- 2 avocados, halved, pitted, and peeled
- 3 tablespoons lime juice, plus more to taste
- 2 small plum tomatoes, diced
- ½ cup finely diced onions
- 2 small cloves garlic, smashed to a paste
- 3 tablespoons chopped fresh cilantro leaves
- ½ scant teaspoon acceptable sea salt
- ½ scant teaspoon ground cumin
- 2 small onions (about 1½-inches in diameter), cut into ½-inch-thick slices
- 8 slices prosciutto

1. Make the guacamole: Place the avocados and lime juice in a large bowl and mash with a fork until it reaches your desired consistency. Add the tomatoes, onions, garlic, cilantro, salt, and cumin, and stir until well combined. Taste and add more lime juice if desired. Set aside half of the guacamole for serving. (Note: If you're making the guacamole ahead of time, place it in a large resealable plastic bag, squeeze out all the air, and seal it shut. It will keep in the refrigerator for up to 3 days when stored this way.)

2. Place a piece of parchment paper on a tray that fits in your freezer and place the onion slices on it, breaking the slices apart into 8 rings. Fill each ring with about 2 tablespoons of guacamole. Place the tray in the freezer for 2 hours.

3.nSpray the air fryer basket with avocado oil. Preheat the air fryer to 400°F (205ºC).

4. Remove the rings from the freezer and wrap each in a slice of prosciutto. Place them in the air fryer basket,

leaving space between them (if you're using a smaller air fryer, work in batches if necessary), and cook for 6 minutes, flipping halfway through. Use a spatula to remove the rings from the air fryer. Serve with the reserved half of the guacamole.

5. Store leftovers in an airtight container in the refrigerator for up to 4 days. Reheat in a preheated 400°F (205ºC) air fryer for about 3 minutes, until heated through.

Per Serving: calories: 132 | fat: 9g | protein: 5g | carbs: 10g | net carbs: 6g | fiber: 4g

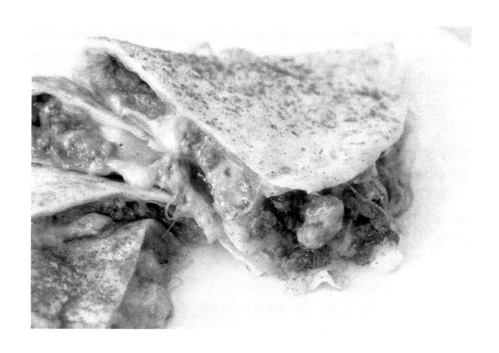

25.Cheesy Pork Rind Tortillas

Prep Time:10 m | **Cook time:**5 m | **Makes** 4

- 1 ounce (28 g) pork rinds
- ¾ cup shredded Mozzarella cheese
- 2 tablespoons full-fat cream cheese
- 1 large egg

1. Place pork rinds into the food processor and pulse until finely ground.
2. Place Mozzarella into a large microwave-safe bowl. Break cream cheese into small pieces and add them to the bowl. Microwave for 30 seconds, or until both kinds of cheese are melted and can easily be stirred together into a ball. Add ground pork rinds and egg to the cheese mixture.
3. Continue stirring until the mixture forms a ball. If it cools too much and cheese hardens, microwave for 10 more seconds.
4. Separate the dough into four small balls. Place each ball of dough between two sheets of parchment and roll into a ¼-inch flat layer.
5. Place tortillas into the air fryer basket in a single layer, working in batches if necessary.
6. Adjust the temperature to 400°F (205ºC) and set the timer for 5 minutes.
7. Tortillas will be crispy and firm when fully cooked.

Per Serving: calories: 145 | fat: 10g | protein: 11g | carbs: 1g | net carbs: 1g | fiber: 0g

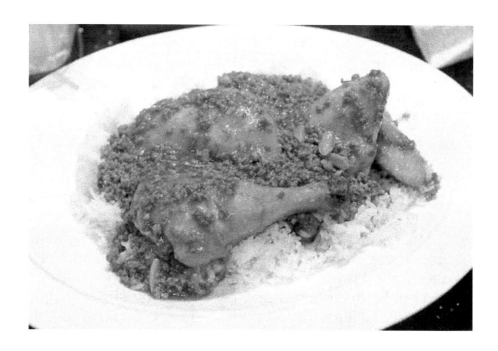

26.Cheesy Pork and Chicken

Prep Time:5 m | **Cook time:**5 m | **Serves:** 2

- 1 ounce (28 g) pork rinds
- 4 ounces (113 g) shredded cooked chicken
- ½ cup shredded Monterey jack cheese ¼ cup sliced pickled jalapeños
- ¼ cup guacamole
- ¼ cup full-fat sour cream

1. Place pork rinds into a 6-inch round baking pan. Cover with shredded chicken and Monterey jack cheese. Place pan into the air fryer basket.
2. Adjust the temperature to 370°F (188°C) and set the timer for 5 minutes or until the cheese is melted.
3. Top with jalapeños, guacamole, and sour cream.

Per Serving: calories: 395 | fat: 27g | protein: 30g | carbs: 3g | net carbs: 2g | fiber: 1g

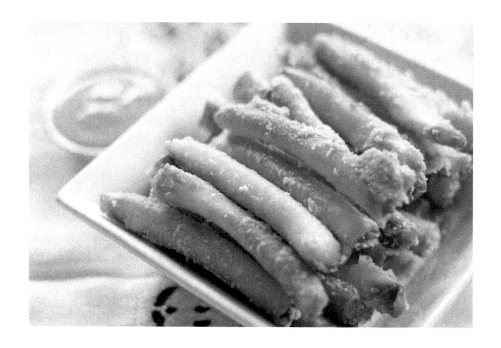

27.Pork Cheese Sticks

Prep Time:20 m | **Cook time:**10 m | Makes 12 sticks

- 6 (1-ounce / 28-g) Mozzarella string cheese sticks
- ½ cup grated Parmesan cheese
- ½ ounce (14 g) pork rinds, finely ground
- 1 teaspoon dried parsley
- 2 large eggs

1. Place Mozzarella sticks on a cutting board and cut them in half. Freeze 45 minutes or until firm. If freezing overnight, remove frozen sticks after 1 hour and place them into an airtight zip-top storage bag and place them back in the freezer for future use.
2. In a large bowl, mix Parmesan, ground pork rinds, and parsley.
3. In a medium bowl, whisk eggs.
4. Dip a frozen Mozzarella stick into beaten eggs and then into a Parmesan mixture to coat. Repeat with the remaining sticks. Place Mozzarella sticks into the air fryer basket.
5. Adjust the temperature to 400°F (205ºC) and set the timer for 10 minutes or until golden.

Per Serving: calories: 236 | fat: 13g | protein: 19g | carbs: 5g | net carbs: 5g | fiber: 0g

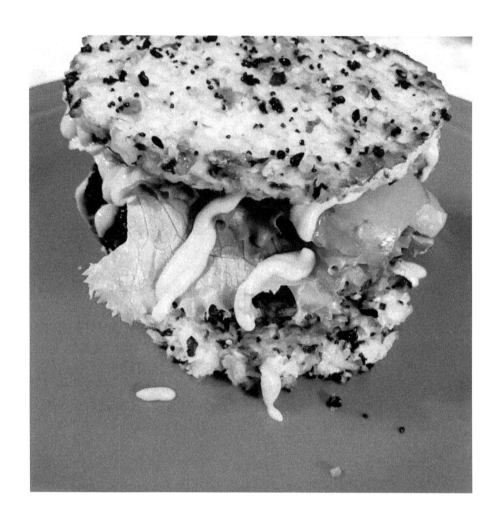

28. Cheesy Cauliflower Buns

Prep Time: 15 m | **Cook time:** 12 m | Makes 8 buns

- 1 (12-ounce 340-g) steamer bag cauliflower, cooked according to package instructions
- ½ cup shredded Mozzarella cheese
- ¼ cup shredded mild Cheddar
- ¼ cup blanched almond flour 1 large egg
- ½ teaspoon salt

1. Let cooked cauliflower cool for about 10 minutes. Use a kitchen towel to wring out excess moisture, then place cauliflower in a food processor.
2. Add Mozzarella, Cheddar, flour, egg, and salt to the food processor and pulse twenty times until the mixture is combined. It will resemble a soft, wet dough.
3. Divide mixture into eight piles. Wet your hands with water to prevent sticking, then press each pile into a flat bun shape, about ½-inch thick.
4. Cut a sheet of parchment to fit the air fryer basket. Working in batches if needed, place the formed dough onto ungreased parchment in an air fryer basket. Adjust the temperature to 350°F (180ºC) and set the timer for 12 minutes, turning buns halfway through cooking.
5. Let buns cool 10 minutes before serving. Serve warm.

Per Serving: calories: 75 | fat: 5g | protein: 5g | carbs: 3g | net carbs: 2g | fiber: 1g

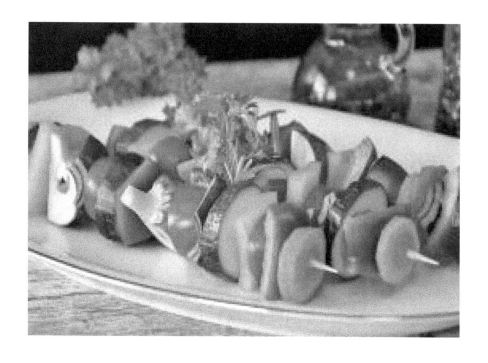

29.Bacon Cauliflower Skewers

Prep Time:10 m | **Cook time:**12 m | **Serves:** 4

- 4 slices sugar-free bacon, cut into thirds
- ¼ medium yellow onion, peeled and cut into 1-inch pieces
- 4 ounces (113 g) (about 8) cauliflower florets 1½ tablespoons olive oil
- ¼ teaspoon salt
- ¼ teaspoon garlic powder

1. Place 1 piece of bacon and 2 pieces of onion on a 6-inch skewer. Add a second piece of bacon, and 2 cauliflower florets, followed by another piece of bacon onto a skewer. Repeat with remaining ingredients and three additional skewers to make four total skewers.
2. Drizzle skewers with olive oil, then sprinkle with salt and garlic powder. Place skewers into an ungreased air fryer basket. Adjust the temperature to 375°F (190ºC) and set the timer for 12 minutes, turning the skewers halfway through cooking. When done, vegetables will be tender, and bacon will be crispy. Serve warm.

Per Serving: calories: 69 | fat: 5g | protein: 5g | carbs: 2g | net carbs: 1g | fiber: 1g

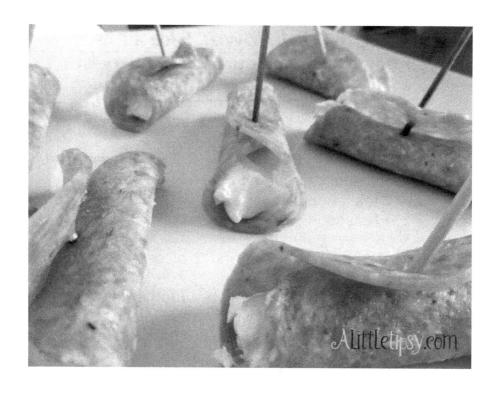

30.Crispy Cheese Salami Roll-Ups

Prep Time:5 m | **Cook time:**4 m | Makes 16 roll-ups

- 4 ounces (113 g) cream cheese, broken into 16 equal pieces
- 16 (0.5-ounce / 14-g) deli slices Genoa salami

1. Place a piece of cream cheese at the edge of a slice of salami and roll to close. Secure with a toothpick. Repeat with remaining cream cheese pieces and salami.
2. Place roll-ups in an ungreased 6-inch round nonstick baking dish and place them into an air fryer basket. Adjust the temperature to 350°F (180ºC) and set the timer for 4 minutes. Salami will be crispy, and cream cheese will be warm when done.

Per Serving: calories: 269 | fat: 22g | protein: 11g | carbs: 2g | net carbs: 2g | fiber: 0g

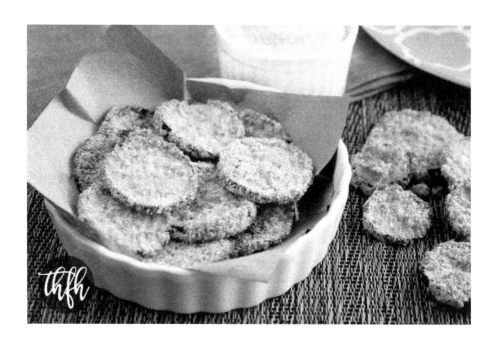

31. Cheesy Zucchini Fries

Prep Time: 10 m | **Cook time:** 10 m | **Serves:** 8

- 2 medium zucchini, ends removed, quartered lengthwise, and sliced into 3-inch long fries
- ½ teaspoon salt
- ⅓ cup heavy whipping cream
- ½ cup blanched finely ground almond flour ¾ cup grated Parmesan cheese
- 1 teaspoon Italian seasoning

1. Sprinkle zucchini with salt and wrap in a kitchen towel to draw out excess moisture. Let sit for 2 hours.
2. Pour cream into a medium bowl. In a separate medium bowl, whisk together flour, Parmesan, and Italian seasoning.
3. Place each zucchini fry into cream, then gently shake off excess. Press each fry into a dry mixture, coating each side, then place into an ungreased air fryer basket. Adjust the temperature to 400°F (205°C) and set the timer for 10 minutes, turning fries halfway through cooking. The fries will be golden and crispy when done. Place on a clean parchment sheet to cool 5 minutes before serving.

Per Serving: calories: 124 | fat: 10g | protein: 5g | carbs: 4g | net carbs: 3g | fiber: 1g

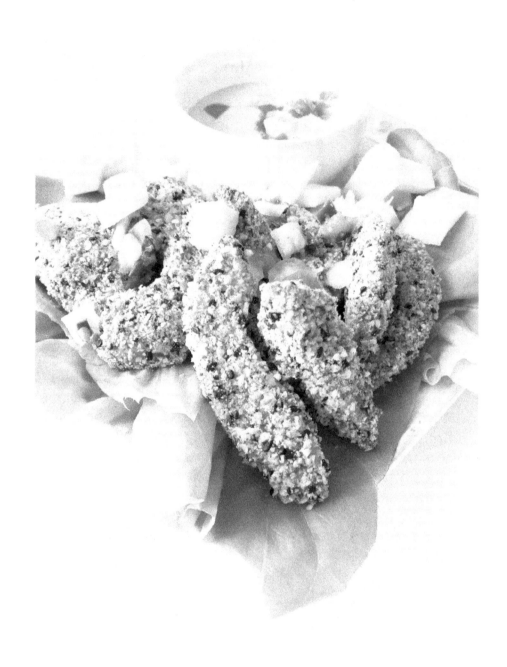

32.Aromatic Avocado Fries

Prep Time:10 m | **Cook time:**15 m | **Serves:** 6

- 3 firm, barely ripe avocados, halved, peeled, and pitted
- 2 cups pork dust (or powdered Parmesan cheese for vegetarian;)
- 2 teaspoons acceptable sea salt
- 2 teaspoons ground black pepper
- 2 teaspoons ground cumin
- 1 teaspoon chili powder
- 1 teaspoon paprika
- ½ teaspoon garlic powder
- ½ teaspoon onion powder
- 2 large eggs
- Salsa, for serving (optional)
- Freshly chopped cilantro leaves for garnish (optional)

1. Spray the air fryer basket with avocado oil. Preheat the air fryer to 400°F (205ºC).
2. Slice the avocados into thick-cut french fry shapes.
3. In a bowl, mix the pork dust, salt, pepper, and seasonings.
4. In a separate shallow bowl, beat the eggs.
5. Dip the avocado fries into the beaten eggs, shake off any excess, and then dip them into the pork dust mixture. Use your hands to press the breading into each fry.
6. Spray the fries with avocado oil and place them in the air fryer basket in a single layer, leaving space between them; if there are too many fries to fit in a single layer, work in batches. Cook in the air fryer for 13 to 15 minutes, until golden brown, flipping after 5 minutes.
7. Serve with salsa, if desired, and garnish with fresh chopped cilantro, if desired. Best served fresh.

8. Store leftovers in an airtight container in the fridge for up to 5 days. Reheat in a preheated 400°F (205°C) air fryer for 3 minutes or until heated through.

Per Serving: calories: 282 | fat: 22g | protein: 15g | carbs: 9g | net carbs: 2g | fiber: 7g

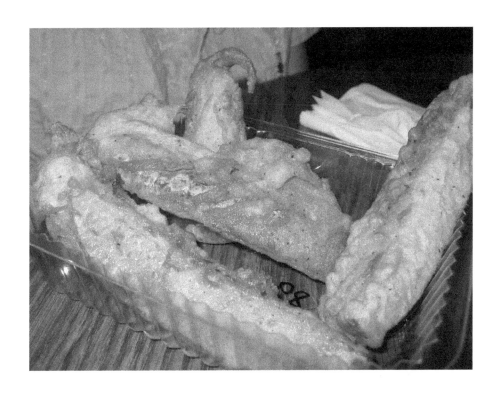

33.Cheesy Pickle Spear

Prep time: 40 m | **Cook time:**10 m | **Serves:** 4

- 4 dill pickle spears, halved lengthwise
- ¼ cup ranch dressing
- ½ cup blanched finely ground almond flour
- ½ cup grated Parmesan cheese
- 2 tablespoons dry ranch seasoning

1. Wrap spears in a kitchen towel for 30 minutes to soak up excess pickle juice.
2. Pour ranch dressing into a medium bowl and add pickle spears. In a separate medium bowl, mix flour, Parmesan, and ranch seasoning.
3. Remove each spear from ranch dressing and shake off excess. Press gently into dry mixture to coat all sides. Place spears into an ungreased air fryer basket. Adjust the temperature to 400°F (205ºC) and set the timer for 10 minutes, turning spears three times during cooking.

Per Serving: calories: 160 | fat: 11g | protein: 7g | carbs: 8g | net carbs: 6g | fiber: 2g

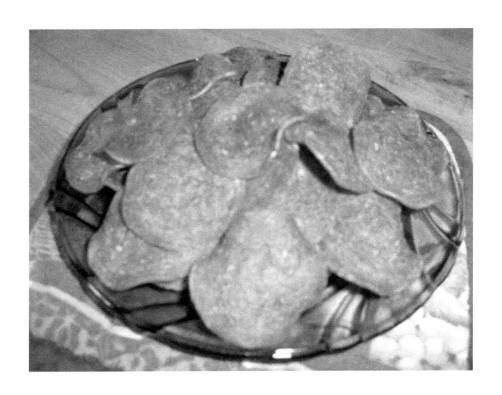

34.Crispy Pepperoni Chips

Prep time: 5 m | **Cook time:**8 m | **Serves:** 2

- 14 slices pepperoni

1.Place pepperoni slices into an ungreased air fryer basket. Adjust the temperature to 350°F (180ºC) and set the timer for 8 minutes. Pepperoni will be browned and crispy when done. Let cool 5 minutes before serving. Store in an airtight container at room temperature for up to 3 days.

Per Serving: calories: 69 | fat: 5g | protein: 3g | carbs: 0g | net carbs: 0g | fiber: 0g

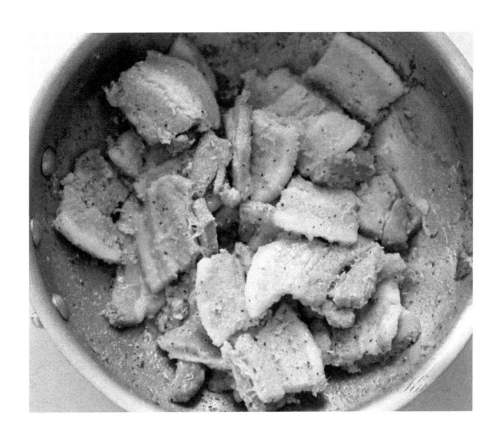

35.Vinegary Pork Belly Chips

Prep Time:5 m | **Cook time:**12 m | **Serves:** 4

- 1 pound (454 g) slab pork belly
- ½ cup apple cider vinegar Fine sea salt
- FOR SERVING (OPTIONAL): Guacamole
- Pico de gallo

1. Slice the pork belly into ⅛-inch-thick strips and place them in a shallow dish. Pour in the vinegar and stir to coat the pork belly. Place in the fridge to marinate for 30 minutes.
2. Spray the air fryer basket with avocado oil. Preheat the air fryer to 400°F (205ºC).
3. Remove the pork belly from the vinegar and place the air fryer basket's strips in a single layer, leaving space between them. Cook in the air fryer for 10 to 12 minutes, until crispy, flipping after 5 minutes. Remove from the air fryer and sprinkle with salt. Serve with guacamole and pico de gallo, if desired.
4. Best served fresh. Store leftovers in an airtight container in the fridge for up to 5 days. Reheat in a preheated 400°F (205ºC) air fryer for 5 minutes, or until heated through, flipping halfway through.

Per Serving: calories: 240 | fat: 21g | protein: 13g | carbs: 0g | net carbs: 0g | fiber: 0g

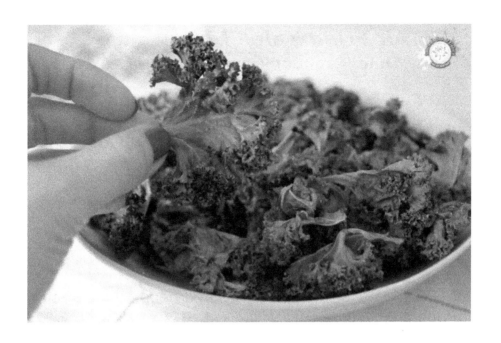

36.Air Fried Kale Chips

Prep Time:5 m | **Cook time:**10 m | Makes 8 cups

- ½ teaspoon dried chives
- ½ teaspoon dried dill weed
- ½ teaspoon dried parsley ¼ teaspoon garlic powder ¼ teaspoon onion powder ⅛ teaspoon acceptable sea salt
- ⅛ teaspoon ground black pepper 2 large bunches of kale

1. Spray the air fryer basket with avocado oil. Preheat the air fryer to 360°F (182ºC).
2. Place the seasonings, salt, and pepper in a small bowl and mix well.
3.Wash the kale and pat completely dry. Use a sharp knife to carve out the thick inner stems, spray the leaves with avocado oil, and sprinkle them with the seasoning mix.
4. Place the kale leaves in the air fryer in a single layer and cook for 10 minutes, shaking and rotating the chips halfway through. Transfer the baked chips to a baking sheet to cool completely and crisp up. Repeat with the remaining kale. Sprinkle the cooled chips with salt before serving, if desired.
5. Kale chips can be stored in an airtight container at room temperature for up to 1 week, but they are best eaten within 3 days.

Per Serving: calories: 11 | fat: 1g | protein: 1g | carbs: 2g | net carbs: 1g | fiber: 1g

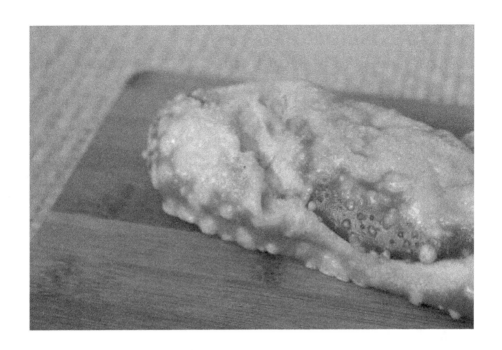

37.Prosciutto Pierogi

Prep Time:15 m | **Cook time:**20 m | **Makes** 4 pierogi

- 1 cup chopped cauliflower
- 2 tablespoons diced onions
- 1 tablespoon unsalted butter (or lard or bacon fat for dairy-free), melted pinch of acceptable sea salt
- ½ cup shredded sharp Cheddar cheese (about 2 ounces / 57 g) (or Kite Hill brand cream cheese style spread, softened, for dairy-free)
- 8 slices prosciutto
- Fresh oregano leaves for garnish (optional)

1. Preheat the air fryer to 350°F (180ºC). Lightly grease a 7-inch pie pan or a casserole dish that will fit in your air fryer.
2. Make the filling: Place the cauliflower and onion in the pan. Drizzle with the melted butter and sprinkle with the salt. Using your hands, mix everything, making sure the cauliflower is coated in the butter.
3. Place the cauliflower mixture in the air fryer and cook for 10 minutes, until fork-tender, stirring halfway through.
4. Transfer the cauliflower mixture to a food processor or high-powered blender. Spray the air fryer basket with avocado oil and increase the air fryer temperature to 400°F (205ºC).
5. Pulse the cauliflower mixture in the food processor until smooth. Stir in the cheese.
6. Assemble the pierogi: Lay 1 slice of prosciutto on a sheet of parchment paper with a short end toward you. Lay another slice of prosciutto on top of it at a right angle, forming a cross. Spoon about 2 heaping tablespoons of the filling into the center of the cross.
7. Fold each arm of the prosciutto cross over the filling to form a square, ensuring that the filling is well covered.

Using your fingers, press down around the filling to even out the square shape. Repeat with the rest of the prosciutto and filling.

8. Spray the pierogi with avocado oil and place them in the air fryer basket. Cook for 10 minutes, or until crispy.

9. Garnish with oregano before serving, if desired. Store leftovers in an airtight container in the fridge for up to 4 days. Reheat in a preheated 400°F (205ºC) air fryer for 3 minutes or until heated through.

Per Serving: calories: 150 | fat: 11g | protein: 11g | carbs: 2g | net carbs: 1g | fiber: 1g

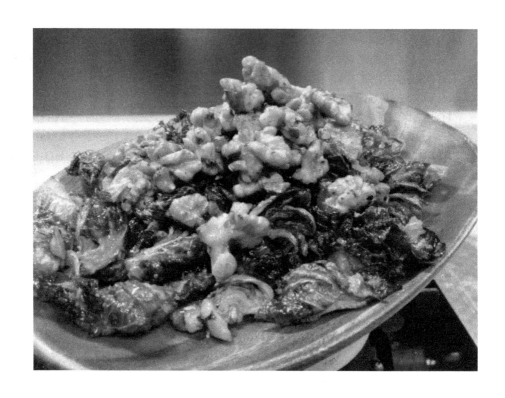

38.Air Fried Brussels Sprout

Prep time: 20 m | **Cook time:**15 m | **Serves:** 4

- 1 pound (454 g) Brussels sprouts, ends, and yellow leaves removed and halved lengthwise
- Salt and black pepper, to taste
- 1 tablespoon toasted sesame oil
- 1 teaspoon fennel seeds
- Chopped fresh parsley for garnish

1. Place the Brussels sprouts, salt, pepper, sesame oil, and fennel seeds in a resealable plastic bag. Seal the bag and shake to coat.
2. Air-fry at 380 degrees F (193ºC) for 15 minutes or until tender. Make sure to flip them over halfway through the cooking time.
3.Serve sprinkled with fresh parsley. Bon appétit!
Per Serving: calories: 174 | fat: 3g | protein: 3g | carbs: 9g | net carbs: 5g | fiber: 4g

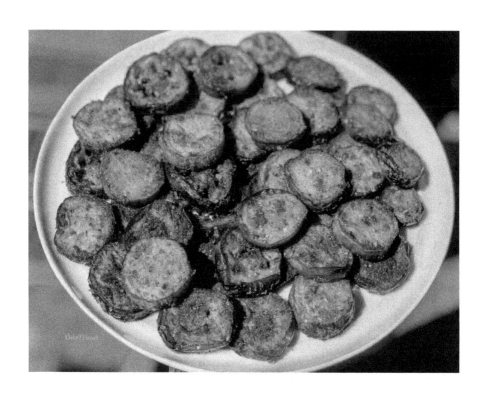

39.Savory Eggplant

Prep Time:45 m | **Cook time:**13 m | **Serves:** 4

- 1 eggplant, peeled and thinly sliced
- Salt, to taste
- ½ cup almond meal ¼ cup olive oil
- ½ cup water
- 1 teaspoon garlic powder
- ½ teaspoon dried dill weed
- ½ teaspoon ground black pepper, to taste

1. Salt the eggplant slices and let them stay for about 30 minutes. Squeeze the eggplant slices and rinse them under cold running water.
2. Toss the eggplant slices with the other ingredients. Cook at 390 degrees F (199ºC) for 13 minutes, working in batches.

Per Serving: calories: 241 | fat: 21g | protein: 4g | carbs: 9g | net carbs: 4g | fiber: 5g

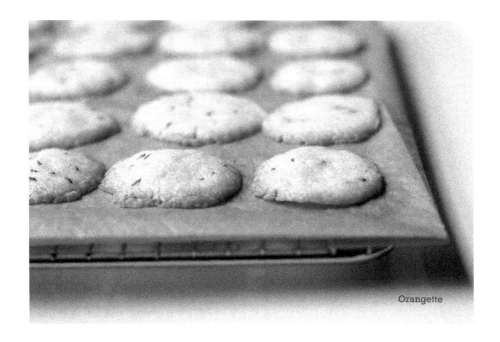

Orangette

40.Golden Cheese Crisps

Prep Time:10 m | **Cook time:**12 m | **Serves:** 2

- ½ cup shredded Cheddar cheese
- 1 egg white

1. Preheat the air fryer to 400°F (205ºC). Place a piece of parchment paper in the bottom of the air fryer basket.
2. In a medium-size bowl, mix the cheese and egg white, stirring with a fork until thoroughly combined.
3. Place small scoops of the cheese mixture in a single layer in the basket of the air fryer (about 1-inch apart). Use the fork to spread the mixture as thin as possible. Air fry for 10 to 12 minutes until the crisps are golden brown. Let cool for a few minutes before transferring them to a plate. Store at room temperature in an airtight container for up to 3 days.

Per Serving: calories: 120 | fat: 10g | protein: 9g | carbs: 1g | net carbs: 1g | fiber: 0g

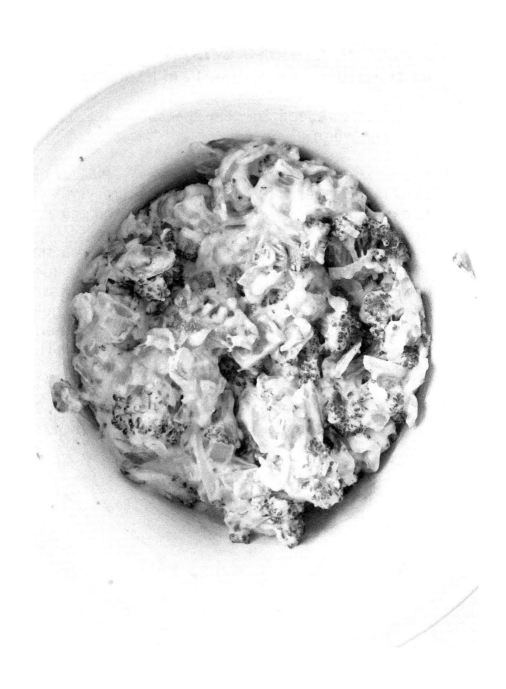

41.Broccoli Fries with Spicy Dip

Prep Time:15 m | **Cook time:**6 m | **Serves:** 4

- ¾ pound (340g) broccoli florets ½ teaspoon onion powder
- 1 teaspoon granulated garlic ½ teaspoon cayenne pepper
- Sea salt and ground black pepper, to taste 2 tablespoons sesame oil
- 4 tablespoons Parmesan cheese, preferably freshly grated Spicy Dip:
- ¼ cup mayonnaise ¼ cup Greek yogurt
- ¼ teaspoon Dijon mustard 1 teaspoon keto hot sauce

1. Start by preheating the Air Fryer to 400 degrees.
2.Blanch the broccoli in salted boiling water until al dente, about 3 to 4 minutes. Drain well and transfer to the lightly greased Air Fryer basket.
3. Add the onion powder, garlic, cayenne pepper, salt, black pepper, sesame oil, and Parmesan cheese.
4. Cook for 6 minutes, tossing halfway through the cooking time.
5. Meanwhile, mix all of the spicy dip ingredients. Serve broccoli fries with chilled dipping sauce. Bon appétit!

Per Serving: calories: 219 | fat: 19g | protein: 5g | carbs: 9g | net carbs: 6g | fiber: 3g

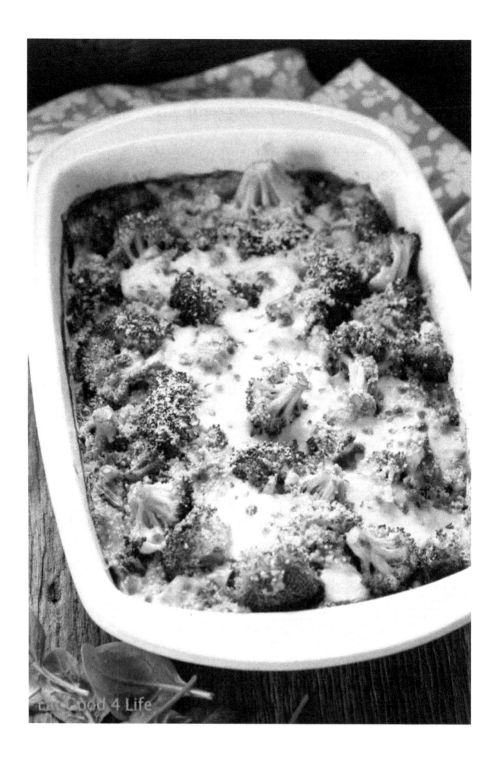

42.Cheesy Broccoli

Prep Time:20 m | **Cook time:**20 m | **Serves:** 6

- 2 eggs, well whisked
- 2 cups Colby cheese, shredded
- ½ cup almond meal
- 2 tablespoons sesame seeds
- Seasoned salt, to taste
- ¼ teaspoon ground black pepper, or more to taste
- 1 head broccoli, grated
- 1 cup Parmesan cheese, grated

1. Thoroughly combine the eggs, Colby cheese, almond meal, sesame seeds, salt, black pepper, and broccoli to make a dough consistency.
2. Chill for 1 hour and shape into small balls; roll the patties over Parmesan cheese. Spritz them with cooking oil on all sides.
3. Cook at 360 degrees F (182ºC) for 10 minutes. Check for doneness and return to the Air Fryer for 8 to 10 more minutes. Serve with a sauce for dipping. Bon appétit!

Per Serving: calories: 322 | fat: 23g | protein: 19g | carbs: 9g | net carbs: 6g | fiber: 3g

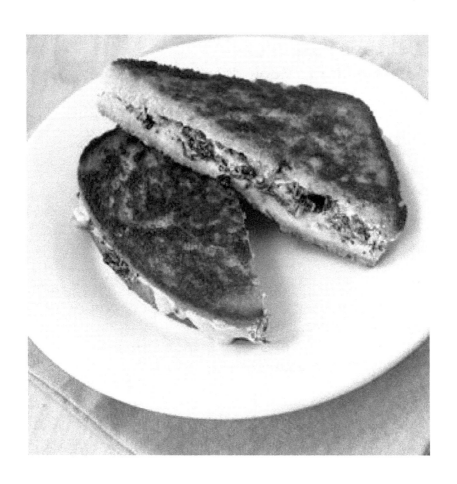

43.Spinach Melts with Chilled Sauce

Prep time: 20 m | **Cook time:** 14 m | **Serves:** 4

Spinach Melts:
- 2 cups spinach, torn into pieces
- 1 ½ cups cauliflower
- 1 tablespoon sesame oil
- ½ cup scallions, chopped
- 2 garlic cloves, minced
- ½ cup almond flour
- ¼ cup coconut flour
- 1 teaspoon baking powder
- ½ teaspoon sea salt
- ½ teaspoon ground black pepper ¼ teaspoon dried dill
- ½ teaspoon dried basil
- 1 cup Cheddar cheese, shredded

Parsley Yogurt Dip:
- ½ cup Greek-Style yogurt
- 2 tablespoons mayonnaise
- 2 tablespoons fresh parsley, chopped
- 1 tablespoon fresh lemon juice
- ½ teaspoon garlic smashed

1. Place spinach in a mixing dish; pour in hot water. Drain and rinse well.
2. Add cauliflower to the steamer basket; steam until the cauliflower is tender, about 5 minutes.
3. Mash the cauliflower; add the remaining ingredients for Spinach Melts and mix to combine well. Shape the mixture into patties and transfer them to the lightly greased cooking basket.
4. Bake at 330 degrees F (166ºC) for 14 minutes or until thoroughly heated.

5. Meanwhile, make your dipping sauce by whisking the remaining ingredients. Place in your refrigerator until ready to serve.
6. Serve the Spinach Melts with the chilled sauce on the side.

Per Serving: calories: 301 | fat: 25g | protein: 11g | carbs: 9g | net carbs: 5g | fiber: 4g

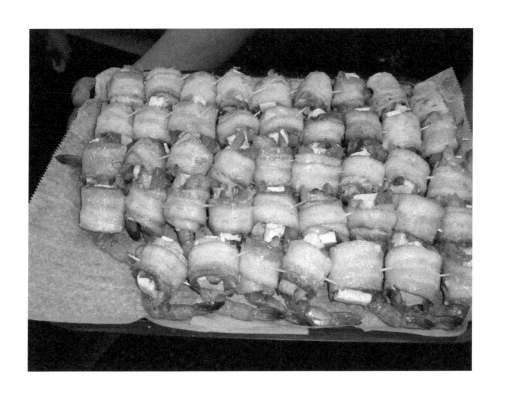

44.Aromatic Bacon Shrimp

Prep time: 45 m | **Cook time:**8 m | **Serves:** 10

- 1¼ pounds (567g) shrimp, peeled and deveined 1 teaspoon paprika
- ½ teaspoon ground black pepper
- ½ teaspoon red pepper flakes, crushed
- 1 tablespoon salt
- 1 teaspoon chili powder
- 1 tablespoon shallot powder ¼ teaspoon cumin powder
- 1¼ pounds (567g) thin bacon slices

1. Toss the shrimps with all the seasoning until they are coated well.
2 Next, wrap a slice of bacon around the shrimps, securing with a toothpick; repeat with the remaining ingredients; chill for 30 minutes.
3. Air-fry them at 360 degrees F (182ºC) for 7 to 8 minutes, working in batches. Serve with cocktail sticks if desired.

Per Serving: calories: 282 | fat: 22g | protein: 19g | carbs: 2g | net carbs: 1g | fiber: 1g

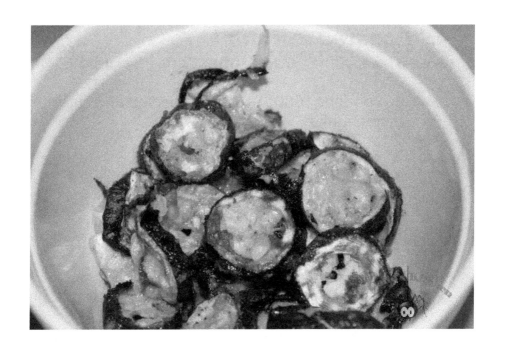

45. Roasted Zucchini

Prep Time: 20 m | **Cook time:** 18 m | **Serves:** 6

- 1½ pounds (680g) zucchini, peeled and cut into ½-inch chunks
- 2 tablespoons melted coconut oil
- A pinch of coarse salt
- A pinch of pepper
- 2 tablespoons sage, finely chopped
- Zest of 1 small-sized lemon
- ⅛ teaspoon ground allspice

1. Toss the squash chunks with the other items.
2. Roast in the Air Fryer cooking basket at 350 degrees F (180°C) for 10 minutes.
3. Pause the machine, turn the temperature to 400 degrees F, stir and roast for an additional 8 minutes.

Per Serving: calories: 270 | fat: 15g | protein: 3g | carbs: 5g | net carbs: 4g | fiber: 1g

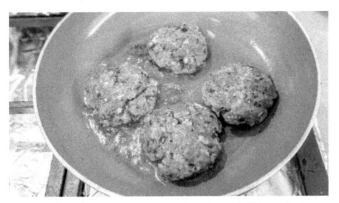

46.Cheesy Meatball

Prep Time:20 m | **Cook time:**18 m | **Serves:** 8

- ½ teaspoon acceptable sea salt
- 1 cup Romano cheese, grated
- 3 cloves garlic, minced
- 1½ pound (680g) ground pork
- ½ cup scallions, finely chopped
- 2 eggs, well whisked
- ⅓ teaspoon cumin powder
- ⅔ teaspoon ground black pepper, or more to taste
  2 teaspoons of basil

1. combine all the ingredients in a large-sized mixing bowl.
2. Shape into bite-sized balls; cook the meatballs in the air fryer for 18 minutes at 345 degrees F (174ºC). Serve with some tangy sauce such as marinara sauce if desired.

Per Serving: calories: 350 | fat: 25g | protein: 28g | carbs: 2g | net carbs: 1g | fiber: 1g

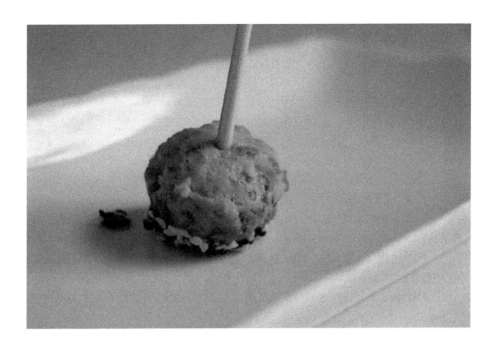

47.Pork Meatball

Prep Time:25 m | **Cook time:**17 m | **Serves:** 8

- 1 teaspoon cayenne pepper
- 2 teaspoons mustard
- 2 tablespoons Brie cheese, grated
- 5 garlic cloves, minced
- 2 small-sized yellow onions, peeled and chopped 1½ pounds (680g) ground pork
- Sea salt and freshly ground black pepper, to taste

1. Mix all of the above ingredients until everything is well incorporated.
2. Now, form the mixture into balls (the size of golf a ball).
3. Cook for 17 minutes at 375 degrees F (190ºC). Serve with your favorite sauce.

Per Serving: calories: 275 | fat: 18g | protein: 3g | carbs: 3g | net carbs: 2g | fiber: 1g

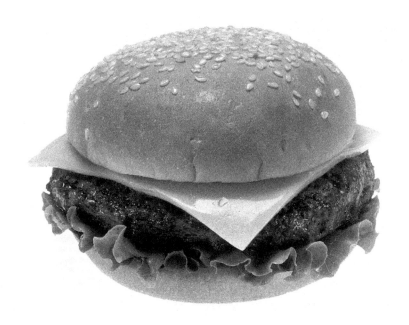

48.Beef Cheese Burger

Prep time: 20 m | **Cook time:**15 m | **Serves:** 4

- 1 tablespoon Dijon mustard
- 2 tablespoons minced scallions
- 1 pound (454 g) ground beef
- 1½ teaspoons minced green garlic
- ½ teaspoon cumin
- Salt and ground black pepper, to taste
- 12 cherry tomatoes
- 12 cubes Cheddar cheese

1. In a large-sized mixing dish, place the mustard, ground beef, cumin, scallions, garlic, salt, and pepper; mix with your hands or a spatula so that everything is evenly coated.
2. Form into 12 meatballs and cook them in the preheated Air Fryer for 15 minutes at 375 degrees F (190ºC). Air-fry until they are cooked in the middle.
3. Thread cherry tomatoes, mini burgers, and cheese on cocktail sticks. Bon appétit!

Per Serving: calories: 469 | fat: 30g | protein: 3g | carbs: 4g | net carbs: 3g | fiber: 1g

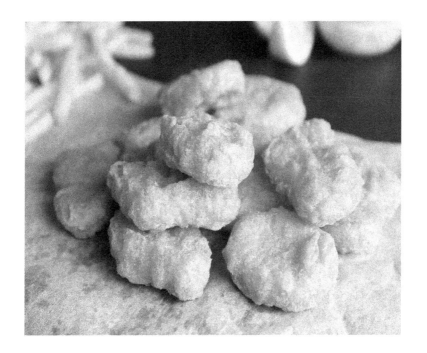

49.Cheesy Chicken Nuggets

Prep Time:20 m | **Cook time:**12 m | **Serves:** 6

- 1 pound (454 g) chicken breasts, sliced into tenders
- ½ teaspoon cayenne pepper Salt and black pepper, to taste ¼ cup almond meal
- 1 egg, whisked
- ½ cup Parmesan cheese, freshly grated ¼ cup mayo
- ¼ cup no-sugar-added barbecue sauce

1. Pat the chicken tenders dry with a kitchen towel. Season with cayenne pepper, salt, and black pepper.
2. Dip the chicken tenders into the almond meal, followed by the egg. Press the chicken tenders into the Parmesan cheese, coating evenly.
3. Place the chicken tenders in the lightly greased Air Fryer basket. Cook at 360 degrees for 9 to 12 minutes, turning them over to cook evenly.
4. In a mixing bowl, thoroughly combine the mayonnaise with the barbecue sauce. Serve the chicken nuggets with the sauce for dipping. Bon appétit!

Per Serving: calories: 268 | fat: 18g | protein: 2g | carbs: 4g | net carbs: 3g | fiber: 1g

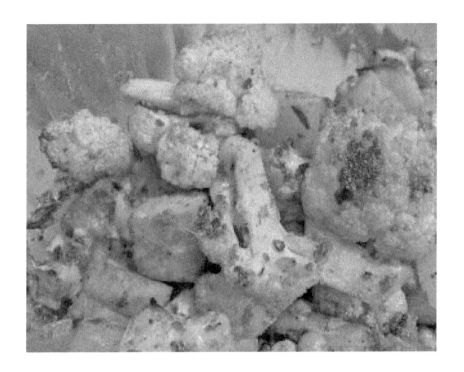

50.Crisp Cauliflower

Prep Time:20 m | **Cook time:**12 m | **Serves:** 2

- 3 cups cauliflower florets
- Two tablespoons sesame oil
- 1 teaspoon onion powder
- 1 teaspoon garlic powder
- 1 teaspoon thyme
- 1 teaspoon sage
- 1 teaspoon rosemary
- Sea salt and cracked black pepper, to taste
- 1 teaspoon paprika

1. Start by preheating your Air Fryer to 400 degrees.
2. Toss the cauliflower with the remaining ingredients; toss to coat well.
3. Cook for 12 minutes, shaking the cooking basket halfway through the cooking time. They will crisp up as they cool. Bon appétit!

Per Serving: calories: 160 | fat: 14g | protein: 3g | carbs: 8g | net carbs: 5g | fiber: 3g